Smart Fat

Cookbook With Fat Meals Which Help You To Lose Weight, Get Healthy And Improve Brain Function

LELA GIBSON

LELA GIBSON

CONTENTS

LELA GIBSON

Introduction

I want to thank you and congratulate you for buying the book, *"Smart Fat"*.

This book contains proven steps and strategies on how to use fat meals to lose weight, get healthy and improve brain function.

For many years, fat has held a bad reputation. Many blamed it for weight gain and various diseases, including stroke and heart attack. Recent research, however, shows that it does not matter that you eat fat- it matters that you eat the right kind of fat. There are many proven benefits to eating the right kinds of fat, often monounsaturated, polyunsaturated, and Omega-3s. These benefits include:

Increased satiety, meaning less hunger cravings and improved weight loss or maintenance efforts

Decreased LDL levels, which lowers the risk of heart disease and stroke

Improved energy levels, especially when the right fats are paired with a low-carb diet

Better absorption of fat-soluble vitamins like A, D, E, and K

Improved brain function from encouraging the production of cell membranes in the brain

This book is filled with recipes that rely on smart fat, the fat that is going to offer all the above benefits. Whether you are eating for your health, to improve brain function, or to lose weight, best of luck with your goals!

Thanks again for buying this book, I hope you enjoy it!

Fat Diet Tips

Despite the many benefits of the fat diet, you may find yourself having a difficult time adjusting to the diet. This is because fat has been demonized for years. In addition, it can be a challenge to actually increase your consumption of fat when you are so much used to eating high-carb foods. However, don't worry because this book will give you some tips to make adopting the diet much easier. Below are some tips that will come in handy as you adopt the smart fat diet:

Start Slow

I am sure you are excited about getting started with the diet; however, go slow. You are not used to eating a lot of fat; thus, you are likely to complain about the taste of food being 'too rich'. This may discourage you from indulging in high-fat foods. Well, it's not a race. You need to give your body some time to adjust.

You can start by slowly increasing your fat intake. Give yourself at least one month to fully embrace the fat diet. Once your body adjusts and starts burning fat, it will be much easier to eat high fat foods.

Use fat to cook

When you start the fat diet, you need to find various opportunities to eat fat. You can start by using it to cook your foods. Instead of steaming or boiling, you should make a habit of frying foods such as vegetables, eggs, fish and meat. Use fats such as butter and other natural fats to fry your food.

Another thing you should note is that different fats bring different flavors to food; thus, you can explore this. Instead of just using the same type of fat to cook, you can change it. You should buy fats such as avocado oil, butter, coconut oil, peanut oil, olive oil, almond oil, macadamia oil, walnut oil, duck fat, lard and tallow. This way, you can discover the various tastes each fat brings to certain foods.

Use full-fat foods

It's not unusual to see foods labeled fat-free, reduced-fat and low-fat. Actually, such foods are often touted to be 'healthier options'. However, you need to forget about such foods. When you're on the fat diet, you need all the fats you get. This means you have to consciously select full-fat products when you do your shopping. Stock your kitchen with foods like eggs and avocados. Select fatty cuts instead of choosing lean cuts of meat. Also, include foods such as sardines and salmon, which tend to contain plenty of healthy fats. Also buy full-fat dairy options. You can also add things such as sour cream or heavy cream. This will boost the amount of fats.

Snack on fat

If you're going to indulge in snacks, you should make sure they are high in fat. You can snack on foods such as boiled eggs, nuts and cheese. Cheese is especially great because it is a great snack. You can use it as an appetizer and you can use it as a topping or dessert.

Sneak fats into your coffee

Yes, you can add fat into your coffee or tea. Fats such as coconut oil and butter are easy to mix in and they give off a warm, comforting taste that is sure to keep you full until it is time for your next meal. However, you'll do well not to misuse this trick. It is easy to overindulge when something tastes good. However, you need to remember that the purpose of eating fats is to give your body the energy it needs. Thus, you should only drink enough to hold you until the next meal.

Fat for weight loss? Not so fast!

Yes, eating fat helps you lose weight. Nevertheless, the reason you want to lose weight in the first place is because you already have excess stored fat. Thus, as you start the fat diet, you should aim at eating just enough fat to avoid feeling hungry. This will allow your body to utilize its internal fat stores.

However, if you are quite hungry, snack on a high fat snack instead of reaching for high-carb snacks. As your body adjusts, you can increase your fat consumption according to your energy needs. Don't make a habit of eating more fats than your body needs. If you've reached the amount if calories you need for the day, give eating a rest.

Garnish and top with fats

Another way you can increase your consumption of fats is by garnishing and topping your food with fats. You can drizzle oil on most foods. You can add fat to the dressing and you can add it to things such as mayo, sour cream and even butter. The important thing is to find ways to increase the amount of fat you eat each day.

You should also make it a point to garnish your meals with foods that have plenty of fats. You can use foods such as avocado, olives, nuts and cheese.

Eat Low-Carb Foods

When you're on the fat diet, your main source of energy should be fats. This means that other sources of energy such as carbohydrates should not be your main source of energy. The thing you should note is that your body is very quick to turn carbs into glucose and use it as fuel. Thus, you should make it a point to eat low-carb foods. This also goes for your snacks. Instead of eating high-carb snacks and desserts, stick to eating high fat snacks and desserts. This way, your body will turn to burning fat.

Fat diets get good reviews for good reasons. They can help you lose weight, improve mental function and increase energy levels. But, before you get any such benefits, you need to take steps to increase your fat consumption. These tips will help you do just that. The following chapters will focus on some high-fat recipes that you can try out that will actually help you lose weight without having to starve yourself.

Breakfast Recipes

Coconut-Raisin Quinoa

Quinoa is a food that can be sweet or savory. In this dish, plump raisins and coconut make it sweet while lime zest and cilantro add a savory touch. A dressing keeps the quinoa moist and tender.

Ingredients

Servings: 4

For the quinoa:

1 cup quinoa (well rinsed)

¼ cup raisins

¼ cup unsweetened coconut

1 ¾ cups water

1 tablespoon coconut oil

¼ cup cilantro (minced)

Zest of one lime

For the dressing:

2 tablespoons grape seed oil (or canola oil)

2 tablespoons lime juice

¾ teaspoon honey

¼ teaspoon salt

Pinch of pepper

Instructions

Add the coconut oil to a small pot over medium heat. When warmed, at the quinoa and allow it to toast for 3-4 minutes, until it begins to stick to the pot. Then, the added water and salt to the pot and turn up the heat. Bring the quinoa to a boil and then set to a simmer, cooking for about 20 minutes until the quinoa is fluffy and the liquid is absorbed.

Use a fork to fluff the quinoa and then mix in the coconut flakes and lime zest. Partially cover the quinoa and allow it to sit an additional 10 minutes before transferring to a bowl. Set the bowl at room temperature until cooled.

While you are waiting, whisk the ingredients for the dressing together in a small bowl. You may want to warm the honey slightly if you cannot get it to mix well with the other ingredients. Once cooled, stir in the raisins and cilantro. Drizzle with the dressing and toss to combine.

Barley with Sunflower Seeds and Bananas

This filling breakfast option combines sweet and nutty flavors. The sunflower seeds provide plenty of healthy fat. Since you can make it in the microwave, it is a quick breakfast option that does not skimp on flavor. If you want a softer barley, consider soaking it the night before.

Ingredients

Servings: 2

2/3 cup pearl barley (quick cooking)

1 1/3 cups water

¼ cup unsalted sunflower seeds

2 medium bananas (sliced)

2 teaspoons honey

Instructions

Add the barley and water to a bowl and cook in the microwave on high heat for about 6 minutes, or until done. You may need to adjust this time based on your microwave. Stir the barley and allow it to sit for 2 minutes. When you are ready to eat, top with the sunflower seeds, sliced bananas, and honey.

Cheesy Bacon Quiche

This simple quiche is light, fluffy, and high in the right kinds of fat. A prepared piecrust makes this quick and easy to throw together. You also save time if you use a can of real bacon bits instead of waiting for your bacon to cook before preparing the quiche.

Ingredients

Servings: 6

1 9-inch pie crust (deep dish, unthawed)

1 can (3 ounces) real bacon bits

1 cup half-and-half

4 eggs (lightly beaten)

¾ cup Swiss cheese (shredded)

¼ cup Parmesan cheese (grated)

1 medium onion (chopped)

Instructions

Set the oven to 400 degrees so it can preheat. While you are waiting, add both cheeses, the bacon bits, and the chopped onions to a bowl and mix together. Then, transfer this into the piecrust.

Add the eggs and half-and-half to another bowl and mix together to incorporate. Pour this into the piecrust, covering the bacon-cheese mixture.

Place your prepared quiche in the oven for 15 minutes. Then, reduce the temperature to 350 degrees for 35 more minutes, until the eggs have set and the top of the quiche starts to brown.

Banana Walnut Pancakes

These pancakes have all the deliciousness of banana-nut bread in an easier, breakfast friendly form. They are also a great way to use up your softening bananas before they go bad.

Ingredients

Servings: 3

1 large or 2 small bananas (overripe)

¼ cup walnuts (finely chopped)

1 cup all-purpose flour)

1 egg

1 cup almond milk

3 tablespoons granulated sugar

1 ½ tablespoons butter (melted)

1 tablespoon baking powder

½ teaspoon baking soda

½ teaspoon cinnamon

½ teaspoon nutmeg

½ teaspoon vanilla extract

½ teaspoon salt

Instructions

Add the walnuts, flour, sugar, baking soda and powder, cinnamon, nutmeg, and salt to a large bowl and mix together to incorporate. Then, make a well in the center of the dry mixture.

In a separate bowl, mash the banana. Then, whisk in the melted butter, almond milk, and vanilla extract. Once smooth, whisk in the egg. Pour this into the well you made in the flour mixture and stir to combine, being careful not to over mix.

Add olive oil or cooking spray to a skillet over medium-high heat. Use about ¼ cup of batter to make each pancake. Drop the batter in and tilt the skillet slightly, carefully spreading it around. Cook about 3-4 minutes until the edges become firm and bubbles start to form. Then, flip and cook an additional 2-3 minutes on the other side.

Easy Baked Egg And Avocado Breakfast Bowl

This is a simple, but flavorful recipe. You can serve as recommended in this recipe, or tweak it by adding some of your favorite flavors.

Ingredients

Servings: 4

8 eggs

4 avocados

4 flour or corn tortillas (warmed)

2 limes

1 teaspoon salt

½ teaspoon black pepper

Scallions (optional, sliced for serving)

Cilantro (optional, chopped for serving)

Chilies (optional, sliced for serving)

Instructions

Start by preheating the oven to 450 degrees. Use a sharp knife to cut each avocado in half, carefully removing the pit. Take a spoon and remove about 1 ½ tablespoons of flesh from the avocado, so the opening is large enough that the egg fits in. Cut the limes in half and squeeze each over 2 of the avocado halves, coating with flesh. Sprinkle salt on top and place on a baking tray.

Once all the avocado halves are prepared, break one egg into each. Season with salt and pepper to taste. Be sure to keep the yolk intact, even if some of the white spills over. If you want your avocados presented nicely, consider using a sieve to separate some of the egg white before putting it inside the avocado.

Cook in the preheated oven for 10-12 minutes, until the yolk is runny but the whites are set. Garnish with the toppings and serve with the warmed tortillas.

Bell Pepper Rings With Egg And Cheese

This quick to prepare dish is packed with weight loss promoting ingredients such as apples and kiwi . These are low-carb and low in calories too.

Ingredients

Servings: 2

1/2 medium sweet red pepper

1/4 cup raspberries

2 large eggs (whole)

1/2 kiwi fruit

1/4 small apples

1/4 small bananas

1 teaspoon extra virgin olive oil

1/4 cup shredded mozzarella cheese

Instructions

Cut the pepper into two 1-inch rounds and then put them in a skillet with some oil.

Crack an egg into each ring and cook the pepper and egg mixture for 3-5 minutes until the egg cooks through.

Top with cheese and cover, and let the cheese melt for about 1 minute.

Mix the fruits and serve alongside the pepper rings.

Almond Pancakes

To help promote satiety, add in blueberries, which also promote oral health and are rich in vitamin C. The berries also strengthen your digestive system.

Ingredients

Servings: 4

1/4 cup blueberries, fresh

2 oz. vanilla whey protein

1/3 cup curd creamed cottage cheese

1 teaspoon baking powder

2 tablespoons dry soy flour, whole grain

3 large eggs

¼ cup almond meal flour

Instructions

Mix baking powder, soy flour, protein powder and almond flour. Stir in the cottage cheese and beaten egg.

Heat a large non-stick skillet over medium heat and use canola oil or butter to lightly grease.

Drop the batter onto the skillet, 1/4 cup per pancake. After bubbles start to form flip the pancake and then cook the other side. This should be done in around 2 minutes.

You can serve with blueberries or alternatively add them to the batter before you cook.

Lunch Recipes

Mexican-Inspired Salmon Cilantro Burgers

This salmon patty is much tastier than ground beef and topped with a cilantro-lime mayo that gives it a Southwest kick. Eat this burger alone for lunch or pair with a side for a filling dinner.

Ingredients

Servings: 8

2 pounds salmon fillet (with skin removed and cut into 1-inch pieces)

½ cup dry breadcrumbs

½ cup canola mayonnaise

1 green onion (chopped)

¼ cup + 2 tablespoons cilantro (chopped)

1 small jalapeno pepper (seeded and minced)

¼ cup + 2 tablespoons fresh lime juice

1 teaspoon + ½ teaspoon salt

½ teaspoon + ¼ teaspoon pepper

Cooking spray

Optional for topping:

Sesame seed hamburger buns

Lettuce leaves (1 per burger)

English cucumber slices (3 per burger)

Instructions

Add the mayonnaise, 2 tablespoons of lime juice, 2 tablespoons of cilantro, and ¼ teaspoon each of salt and pepper to a small bowl and whisk to combine. Set this in the fridge to chill while you prepare the burgers.

Add the salmon chunks to a food processor and pulse until it is coarsely chopped. Then, add the remaining ingredients to the processor and pulse until well combined. Form this into 8 patties.

Place a grill pan on the stove and warm it to medium-high heat. Use cooking spray to coat the pan before adding the patties. Cook about 2 minutes on each side, until cooked to your desired level of doneness. Serve the salmon with the mayonnaise mixture on a bun, topping with the lettuce and English cucumbers if you choose.

Crab Cakes

These flavorful patties can be enjoyed as a standalone, as a slider, or as a side to a salad. They make for an easy and delicious lunch and even taste good reheated, so you can make them a couple days ahead of time and grab them for your lunch or a snack throughout the day.

Ingredients

Servings: 8

1 pound fresh lump crab meat

1 can pink salmon (boneless, skinless)

3 eggs

½ cup pork rinds (crushed)

2 tablespoons mayo

2 tablespoons avocado flesh

1 tablespoon lemon juice

1 tablespoon garlic powder

1 tablespoon relish

1 teaspoon salt

Olive oil for frying

Instructions

Add everything except the olive oil to a large bowl and mix to combine. Be cautious of over mixing. Form this into 8 patties and set to the side.

Set a skillet on the stove over medium heat. Add the olive oil and allow to warm before adding the patties, 2 at a time. Cook for about 6 minutes on each side, until the patties are golden brown.

Seared Chicken Breast Halves And Strawberry Avocado Salsa

This dish tastes great on top of the salad and is perfect when strawberries are in season. The recipe does call for jalapeno, which gives this dish a small kick but not much. You can omit them if you choose.

Ingredients

Servings: 4

4 chicken breast halves (about 4 ounces each)

1 medium avocado (diced)

1 ½ cups strawberries (chopped)

2 tablespoons cilantro (chopped)

2 tablespoons jalapeno pepper (seeded and minced)

1 tablespoon olive oil

2 teaspoons lime juice

½ teaspoon + ¼ teaspoon salt

¼ teaspoon pepper

1 lime (cut into 4 wedges, for serving)

Instructions

Add the avocado, strawberries, jalapeno, lime juice, cilantro, and ¼ teaspoon of the salt to a small bowl. Gently but thoroughly mix to combine. Set this to the side.

Place a large skillet on the stove and warm to medium heat. Add the oil and allow it to warm before distributing it around the pan. Then, pat the chicken dry with paper towels and add the remaining salt and the pepper to both sides of each breast. Cook the chicken for about 4-5 minutes on one side and then flip, cooking an additional 4-5 minutes. Cook longer if necessary so the chicken is cooked all the way through.

If you are serving as a salad, prepare the lettuce on the plates. Add one chicken breast half to each plate and top with the strawberry avocado salsa. Garnish with a lime wedge.

Open-Faced Avocado And Salmon

Tender, flaky salmon and creamy avocado top this traditional BLT on a single slice of toasted bread. Creamy, flaky, and crispy ingredients will excite your taste buds. Plus, who doesn't love bacon?

Ingredients

Servings: 4

4 salmon fillets (3/4" thick, about 4 ounces)- with skin removed

4 slices rustic Italian bread

4 slices center-cut bacon

½ avocado (peeled and pitted, cut into 8 slices)

4 tomato slices (1/4-inch thick)

4 lettuce leaves

¼ cup canola mayo

1 ½ teaspoons Dijon mustard

2 tablespoons water

2 teaspoons + 1 teaspoon fresh chives (minced)

½ lemon (cut into 4 wedges, for garnish)

Instructions

Set the broiler on high heat. When heated, place the Italian bread on a baking sheet and broil until toasted, flipping the bread half way through so both sides are browned. This should take about 1 minute on each side.

Then, place the bacon in a nonstick skillet and cook over medium heat. Once crispy, remove it from the pan and set to the side on a rack or a plate with a paper towel. Put the salmon in the pan you cooked the bacon in and cook 8 minutes total, flipping halfway through. You can adjust this cooking time to your desired doneness.

While you are waiting for the salmon to finish cooking, add the mayo, Dijon mustard, water, and 2 teaspoons of the chives to a small bowl and mix thoroughly to incorporate. Spread this mixture on the toasted bread. Then, assemble the sandwiches by adding 1 leaf of lettuce, 1 tomato slice, 1 bacon slice, 1 fish fillet, and 2 slices of avocado to each piece of bread. Sprinkle with the remaining chives and garnish with lemon wedges for serving.

Pesto Zucchini Noodles

Zucchini is a nutrient-dense food high in fiber, a substance that keeps the digestive system working properly. It's also rich in vitamin C and antioxidants which help remove toxins that contribute to weight gain.

Ingredients

Servings: 4

2-3 tablespoons prepared basil pesto

2 cups broccoli florets

1/2 cup green onions cut into 1-inch pieces

6 slices of uncooked bacon

Generous pinch of salt

4 medium zucchini, julienned thinly

Romano or Parmesan cheese, for garnish

Instructions

Put the zucchini in a colander in the sink or over a bowl and then sprinkle with salt; toss to combine. Let the zucchini sit for about 15 minutes then drain the excess water by squeezing the zucchini.

Cook the bacon in a skillet over medium heat, until crisp, as you turn it regularly. Then remove the bacon to paper towels to dry.

Crumble the bacon and remove the bacon drippings; but reserve about 2 tablespoons of the drippings.

Add in the broccoli and the green onions into the pan. Stir frequently and cook over medium heat until crisp tender, in about 3-5 minutes.

Add in 2 tablespoons of pesto and zucchini and toss to combine. Taste and adjust the seasonings as desired and let it heat up for 2-3 minutes.

Top with freshly grated Parmesan cheese and bacon crumbles.

Beef, Scallions And Red Bell Pepper

Lean cuts of beef from organic or grass fed cattle has low saturated fats and is high in quality protein. Protein is an important building block for strong muscles as well as being great for satiety. You can add in peppers and onions for extra flavor.

Ingredients

Servings: 2

1/4 cup mozzarella cheese, shredded

1/2 cup sweet red peppers, chopped

1/4 cup scallions or spring onions, chopped

5 ounce steak

Instructions

Over medium-high heat, sauté beef cut into thin strips in a small skillet for about 1- 2 minutes.

Add red pepper, scallions, and sauté the mixture for the pepper to soften and the beef to become brown. Now add in pepper and salt to taste and drain the extra fat.

Put the meat mixture onto a place and sprinkle the cheese. Let the cheese to melt before serving.

Dinner Recipes

Salmon With Toasted Walnuts And Walnut Sherry Vinaigrette

Healthy fats in this recipe come from walnuts, walnut oil, and omega-3 rich salmon. This can be served over a bed of asparagus, snap peas, or cauliflower rice. It also tastes great on top of a salad.

Ingredients

Servings: 4

4 boneless salmon fillets with skin on (about 1/3 pound each)

½ cup toasted walnut halves (chopped)

1/3 cup shallots (diced)

1/3 cup walnut oil

¼ cup Sherry vinegar

1 tablespoon olive oil

1 teaspoon sugar

Salt and pepper to taste

Instructions

Set the oven to 375 degrees so it can preheat. Place a 9x13 roasting pan until it preheats (do not use glass). While you are waiting, place the salmon with the skin side down on a plate or cutting board and add salt and pepper to taste. Carefully remove the roasting pan and place the salmon skin side down inside of it.

Bake the salmon for 8-10 minutes, until it flakes with a fork. You want to be very careful not to overcook it, because it will become dry very fast.

While you are waiting, place a small skillet on the stove over medium heat. Add the shallots and cook until golden in color and softened, for about 2 minutes. Then, add the sugar and stir until it dissolves. Once dissolved, add the vinegar and some salt and pepper. Cook an additional minute before removing from the stove.

Add the oil and shallot mixture to a medium bowl. Add the walnut oil and whisk until well combined. Then, stir in the walnuts. Once the salmon is cooked, add to a plate and drizzle with the vinaigrette. Serve with your chosen side.

Single-Skillet Seared Avocado And Chicken

Robust, hearty flavors come together in this dish that won't leave every pan in your home dirty. A small amount of sugar is used while searing the avocados to char them and bring out their flavors.

Ingredients

Servings: 4

4 boneless, skinless chicken breast halves (about 6 ounces each)

4 green onions (trimmed)

2 small ripened avocados (cut in half with pits removed)

1/3 cup sour cream

2 medium red onions (cut into ¼" rings)

1 poblano pepper (sliced)

3 tablespoons lime juice

2 tablespoons water

1 tablespoon soy sauce

1 tablespoon olive oil

¼ teaspoon + ¼ teaspoon sea salt

½ teaspoon ancho chili powder

½ teaspoon black pepper

¼ teaspoon sugar

1 lime (cut into 4 wedges, for garnish)

8 sprigs cilantro (for garnish)

Instructions

Set the oven to 450 degrees so it can preheat. Set a large cast iron skillet on the stove and warm to a medium-high temperature. Place the olive oil inside and distribute evenly.

While you are waiting for the olive oil to warm, add the chili powder, pepper, and ¼ teaspoon salt to the chicken. Add to the pan and cook for 4 minutes. Then, flip it and cook another minute. Transfer to a plate (it will not be fully cooked yet).

Carefully wipe the skillet with paper towels to clean it. Add a non-stick cooking spray and turn up the temperature to high heat. Sprinkle the sugar on top of the avocado halves and place them cut side down in the pan. Cook until charred, about 2 minutes. Remove from the skillet and set aside.

Then, spray the pan again and add the red onions. Char on high heat for about 3 minutes and flip, adding the poblano pepper and green onions. Use a fork to separate the rings of the onion and toss with the green onions and poblano. Stir the soy sauce and lime juice into the pan and distribute.

Distribute the chicken breast halves and avocados across the pan and bake for about 7 minutes in the oven, until the chicken is cooked all the way through.

When the chicken is cooked, remove from the oven and let cool slightly. While you are waiting, mix together the sour cream and water in a bowl. Serve the chicken and avocados with the sour cream mixture and top with a lime wedge and 2 sprigs of cilantro each. Sprinkle with remaining salt if you would like.

Crockpot Thai Pork And Peppers With Peanut Sauce

Using a quality nut butter is important to get the healthy fats from this recipe. The peanut sauce and tender pork pairs beautifully. It is even better that this is a low-maintenance crockpot meal that you can throw together and then forget about for a few hours. If you gather the ingredients ahead of time, it takes less time to prepare this than to call for Thai takeout.

Ingredients

Servings: 4

1 pound boneless pork chops

2 red bell peppers (cut into thin slices, then into bite-sized pieces)

6 cloves garlic (minced)

1 cup low-sodium chicken broth

1/3 cup creamy nut butter

1/3 cup soy sauce

3 tablespoons honey

2 tablespoons ginger (minced)

1 teaspoon red pepper flakes

Instructions

Add all the ingredients except the pork chops in the slow cooker and stir to combine. Then, place the pork chops inside and spoon the mixture over them, coating thoroughly. Cook for 5-6 hours on the low heat setting of your crock pot.

Once the pork is tender, carefully remove it from the pot and place it on a cutting board. Use two forks to shred the pork into pieces. Then, return the pork to the crock pot and stir into the sauce. Allow to cook an additional 10-15 minutes while the pork soaks up more of the peanut sauce and serve. You can eat this alone, with a side of white, brown, or cauliflower rice, or with a side of veggies.

Bacon And Cheese Stuffed Chicken Breasts With Lemony Green Beans And Almonds

Tender chicken breasts are filled with goat's cheese and bacon for a salty, creamy experience. The green beans with almonds have a nice, bright flavor in comparison.

Ingredients

Servings: 2

For the chicken:

2 chicken breasts (with or without skin)

¾ cup goats cheese (softened to room temperature)

2 slices bacon (chopped)

1 tablespoon olive oil

½ teaspoon salt

¼ teaspoon pepper

For the green beans:

1 cup green beans (cleaned and trimmed)

Juice of ½ lemon

Zest of ½ lemon

¼ cup almonds (toasted and chopped)

Instructions

Add the bacon to a medium skillet and fry until lightly golden in color. Then, carefully remove the bacon with a slotted spoon and place on a plate lined with a paper towel.

Place the chicken breasts on a cutting board and pat dry with a paper towel. Season them with the salt and pepper and then use a sharp knife to cut down the middle on one side, keeping the inside sealed.

Take the cooled bacon and put it in the bowl with the goats cheese. Mix until incorporated and add extra pepper if you would like. Then, stuff the breasts with this mixture and gently close. You can use a toothpick if you would like.

Bring the olive oil to temperature over medium high heat and add the chicken breasts to the skillet. Cook until the chicken is cooked completely and golden brown, about 4-5 minutes on each side. Set this to the side to rest while you prepare the green beans.

Bring water and a little salt to a boil and put the green beans in the pan for 1-2 minutes. Rinse them with cool water and then drizzle with the lemon juice. Top with the toasted almonds and lemon zest and serve alongside the chicken.

Miso Salmon And Wilted Spinach

This Asian-inspired dish tastes great on top of rice, either white or brown. If you want a lower carb option, you could try cauliflower rice as well.

Ingredients

Servings: 2

For the fish:

2 salmon fillets (about 6 ounces, with skin removed)

1 tablespoon white miso paste

2 teaspoons low-sodium soy sauce

2 teaspoons rice vinegar

2 teaspoons sweet rice wine (mirin)

1 teaspoon toasted sesame seeds

½ teaspoon fresh ginger (grated)

½ teaspoon sugar

For the wilted spinach:

10 ounces (1 package) fresh spinach

1 teaspoon minced garlic

2 teaspoons low-sodium soy sauce

2 teaspoons dark sesame oil

Instructions

Turn on the broiler so it can preheat. Add all the ingredients for the fish except the salmon and sesame seeds to a small bowl. Whisk to incorporate and set to the side.

Prepare a baking tray by lining it with foil. Use a brush to paint the prepared miso mixture on each fillet, making a thick and even coating. Place these in the broiler for about 8 minutes, or until the fish reaches your desired doneness level. When it is done, sprinkle with the toasted sesame seeds before serving.

A couple minutes before the salmon is done, warm the sesame oil to medium-high heat in a large skillet. Add the spinach and garlic and cook until the spinach just starts to wilt, about 30 seconds as you continuously toss the mixture. Then, stir in the soy sauce and remove from heat. Serve alongside the salmon fillets.

Spaghetti Squash & Meatballs

This is an easy to cook and mild flavored spaghetti squash, and can work as a good replacement to pasta. The weight friendly dish only has 42 calories and only 10 grams per cup. Real pasta has whopping 210 calories and 42 grams of carbs per cup!

Ingredients

Servings: 4

1 cup shredded mozzarella cheese

1lb prepared meatballs

1 cup marinara sauce

2 medium-sized spaghetti squash

Salt & pepper

Olive oil

Instructions

Preheat the oven to around 400 degrees F. Use a small, sharp knife to pierce the center of the spaghetti a number of times. Microwave it for around 3 minutes ensuring that you flip it once as it cooks.

Cut the spaghetti squash lengthwise into half, and then use a spoon to remove the seeds.

Onto a baking sheet that is lined with foil, lay the spaghetti halves and then brush with oil; season with salt and pepper.

Roast it until ready, say in 50-60 minutes, and let it cool down for another 10 minutes. As the squash roasts, prepare the meatballs.

As soon as the squash completely cools, use a fork to scrape the flesh to loosen and fluff the strands.

Before serving, top with 1/4 cup shredded mozzarella cheese, 1/4 cup sauce and 4 meatballs. Then broil so that the cheese turns brown and bubbly.

Soup, Side, And Snack Recipes

Tortilla Soup With Avocado And Shrimp

The healthy fats in this delicious soup come from the shrimp and the avocado. It has the perfect blend of smokiness and spiciness to delight your taste buds. You can garnish with cheddar, sour cream, or cilantro in addition to the tortilla strips.

Ingredients

Servings: 4

12 ounces medium-sized shrimp (peeled and deveined, with tails removed)

1 cup avocado (diced)

4 cups low-sodium chicken broth

1 can (15 ounces) fire-roasted diced tomatoes (with juices)

1 can (15 ounces) white hominy (drained and rinsed)

1 ounce tortilla chips (lightly crushed)

1 cup onion (chopped)

1/3 cup carrot (chopped)

1/3 cup celery (chopped)

3 garlic cloves (minced)

1 tablespoon chipotle chili in adobo sauce (minced)

1 tablespoon lime juice

1 tablespoon olive oil

1 teaspoon chili powder

1 teaspoon cumin

Instructions

Place a Dutch oven or a large soup pot on the stove and warm to medium-high heat. Add the olive oil and distribute. Then, add the onion, carrot, celery, garlic, chipotle chili, chili powder, and cumin to the pan. Stir until the carrot starts to become tender, about 6 minutes. Then, add the fire-roasted tomatoes, hominy, and chicken broth. Turn up the heat and bring the mixture to a boil.

Once boiling, cover the pot and cook for 6 minutes. Then, add the shrimp and cook all the way through, about 2 minutes. Take the pan off the stove and add the salt and lime juice. Stir to incorporate. Serve in bowls and top with the avocado and crushed chips, as well as any other toppings you choose.

Apple Walnut Salad

This sweet and savory salad offers a medley of flavors and a medley of healthy fats. Its fat sources include walnuts, cream cheese, and full-fat yogurt. This tastes great alongside chicken or pork and is so tasty you could eat it alone for dessert.

Ingredients

Servings: 8

6 large apples (cored, peeled, and diced)

1 ½ cups + ¼ cup walnuts (chopped)

1 container (6 ounces) full-fat plain yogurt

1 package (8 ounces) cream cheese (softened)

1 cup dried cranberries

¾ cup brown sugar

1 teaspoon vanilla

1 teaspoon cinnamon

Instructions

Mix the brown sugar and cinnamon together in a bowl. Then, add the yogurt, cream cheese, and vanilla and beat until smooth. Stir in the chopped apples, dried cranberries, and 1 ½ cups of walnuts. Mix until everything is thoroughly coated. Place in a bowl and top with the remaining walnuts. Chill 1-2 hours before serving.

Avocado Citrus Salad

This citrus-y salad makes the perfect pairing with chicken, pork, or even fish that is rich in healthy fats. It can also be eaten as a standalone lunch or snack.

Ingredients

Servings: 4

2 avocados (halved, pitted, peeled, and cut into slices)

1 large pink grapefruit

1 head romaine lettuce

2 tablespoons white wine vinegar

4 tablespoons olive oil

1 teaspoon salt

½ teaspoon pepper

Instructions

Take a paring knife (or a zester) and remove 1 tablespoon of zest from the grapefruit, being sure to avoid the white bitter-tasting pith found under the peel. Then, use a sharp knife to cut the grapefruit in half over a medium bowl. Cut into the individual segments of grapefruit by slicing along the membrane on either side, leaving behind the membrane as you work. Set the bowl to the side and reserve the grapefruit rind halves.

Take the vinegar, oil, and salt and pepper and add it to a medium bowl. Whisk it together and then squeeze the grapefruit rinds over the bowl, extracting the remaining juice. Stir in the zest.

Next, put the avocado slices in the bowl and coat with the dressing, spooning it over gently so the avocados remain intact. Gently stir in the grapefruit segments you set to the side. Set this bowl to the side while you roughly chop the romaine lettuce into bite-sized pieces. Serve this on four individual plates and top each with ¼ of the grapefruit and avocado slices and drizzle with the remaining dressing.

White Bean Salad With Bacon, Cheddar, And Walnuts

This savory salad makes a perfect accompaniment to fish, chicken, or pork. It offers healthy fats from the cheddar cheese and walnuts.

Ingredients

Servings: 10

3 can (15 ounces each) white Great Northern beans (drained and rinsed)

4 slices bacon (cooked, cooled, and crumbled)

1 medium red bell pepper (minced)

2 whole garlic heads

½ cup sharp cheddar cheese (shredded)

½ cup toasted walnuts (chopped)

½ cup parsley (chopped)

½ cup celery (chopped)

1/3 cup + 1 teaspoon olive oil

2 tablespoons apple cider vinegar

1 tablespoon Dijon mustard

1 teaspoon salt

½ teaspoon pepper

Instructions

Start by setting the oven to 350 degrees to preheat. Carefully remove the extra skin layers from the garlic, without separating the individual cloves. Then, slice the tips off and set the garlic on a piece of foil. Use the single teaspoon of oil to drizzle the heads and wrap them in the foil. Cook until slightly browned and soft, about an hour. Once the garlic is finished, carefully unwrap it and set it to the side to cool.

When cooled, squeeze the cloves out of their skins and into a food processor. Then, add the remaining oil, along with the mustard, vinegar, and thyme. Puree until smooth before adding the salt and pepper. Then, pulse to combine.

Next, add the beans to a large bowl with the crumbled bacon, toasted walnuts, bell pepper, parsley, and celery. Mix to combine and coat with the dressing. Then, add the cheese and gently stir. You can chill before serving or eat at room temperature.

Healthy Fat Olive Balls

These balls have olives, cream cheese, and pecans, all of which are great sources of healthy fats. These little bites are great for an anytime snack and even work well as an appetizer for parties.

Ingredients

Servings: 25

½ jar (3.5 ounces) green olives (with pimentos)

2 tablespoons juice from the olives

¾ cup pecans (chopped)

1 package (8 ounces) cream cheese (softened)

¼ teaspoon seasoned salt

Instructions

Add the cream cheese, seasoned salt, and 2 tablespoons olive juice to a food processor and pulse until well combined. Transfer to a bowl and place in the refrigerator for about 30 minutes, until it firms.

Once firm, use the mixture to surround each olive. You should have enough mixture to make 12-13 balls. Place the pecans in a shallow bowl or on a plate and roll the balls in them. Place them on a wax-lined tray and return to the refrigerator to firm up. You can then cut in halves if you would like- each ball is 2 servings.

Buttermilk Avocado Soup Topped With Crab Salad

Crab is a good source of Omega-3s and avocados are rich in monounsaturated fats. You can adjust the amount of buttermilk added until your soup achieves a smooth, creamy consistency. This will also cut down on some of the avocado flavor, if you do not want a strong avocado taste.

Ingredients

Servings: 8

For the soup:

4 ripened avocados (pitted and peeled)

1 ½ cups fat-free buttermilk

2 small tomatillos (chopped)

½ cup low-sodium chicken broth

1 large clove garlic

2 serrano peppers (seeded)

3/4 teaspoon salt

For the crab salad:

16 ounces crab meat (drained)

¼ cup red bell pepper (minced)

2 tablespoons chives (chopped)

1 tablespoon lemon juice

1 teaspoon orange zest

Instructions

Add all the ingredients for the soup to a blender. Blend until you have a smooth, creamy consistency. Adjust the buttermilk as needed to meet your preference.

Then, add the crab and other ingredients to a large bowl. Gently toss everything until well combined. Serve the soup in a bowl with the crab salad on top.

Avocado Salsa

This easy to prepare salsa can be served with fish or shellfish dishes, chicken or as a dip. Avocados are full of healthy fats and potassium. The fats help keep you full for longer and are great for fighting off occasional cravings.

Ingredients

Servings: 1

1/8 teaspoon black pepper

1/8 teaspoon salt

1/8 cup cilantro

2 tablespoons fresh lime juice

1 California avocado

1 small red onion

1/2 jalapeno pepper

1 small whole red tomato

Instructions

Chop the cilantro and tomato and set aside, then finely dice the jalapeno pepper and onion.

Remove the skin from the avocado, chop it and place in on a serving bowl. Add in lime juice, jalapeno and the onion. Gently mix the avocado mixture. Add in the cilantro and tomato and mix; season with salt and pepper.

Cover and chill until ready to be served.

I need your help...

Thank you again for buying this book!

I hope this book was able to help you to get an idea about how to use fat meals to lose weight, get healthy and improve brain function.

The next step is to take action.

Finally, if you enjoyed this book, would you be kind enough to leave a review for this book on Amazon?

I want to reach as many people as I can with this book, and more reviews will help me accomplish that!

If you have any questions or problems, please contact us: hello@freedomdestination.com

Thank you and good luck!

Preview Of 'Negative Calorie Diet'

Negative Calorie Diet: What Is It

This unique diet draws upon the idea that some foods have the 'negative calorie' effect that we ought to consider in burning fat. A food is considered to have a negative calorie effect when the calories these foods use to digest are typically higher than the calories in the foods themselves.

When you eat something, you begin by chewing, a process that consumes energy. Some foods such as those higher in stringy fibers like celery will require more chewing, which will result in more energy expenditure, and there are others like pasta and cakes that don't require as much chewing.

After chewing, the foods go to the stomach through the esophagus and the other processes of digestion take over until absorption takes place and the body excretes the residual mass.

With negative calorie foods, this entire process uses up more calories than the foods have. The extra calories the body has to provide in order to process the foods are taken from the fat stores, and the more of these negative calorie foods you eat, the more your fat stores will lose calories, and as a result, the more fat you will lose.

Let us take broccoli as an example: 100 grams (contains 25 calories).

When you eat 100 grams of broccoli, it takes your body about 80 calories worth of energy to digest it. This results in a net calorie use of 55 calories that should come from the fat stores in your body. As you can see, the 55 calories make up the negative net calorie.

Let us now take a counter example of a piece of cake containing 400 calories.

Your body will take about 150 calories to digest the piece of cake, leaving net 250 calories deposited in the body and stored as fat.

The negative calorie diet consists of over 100 foods proven to have negative calorie qualities. Most of these foods are fruits and veggies that are high in fiber. Let us look at them in more detail in the following chapter.

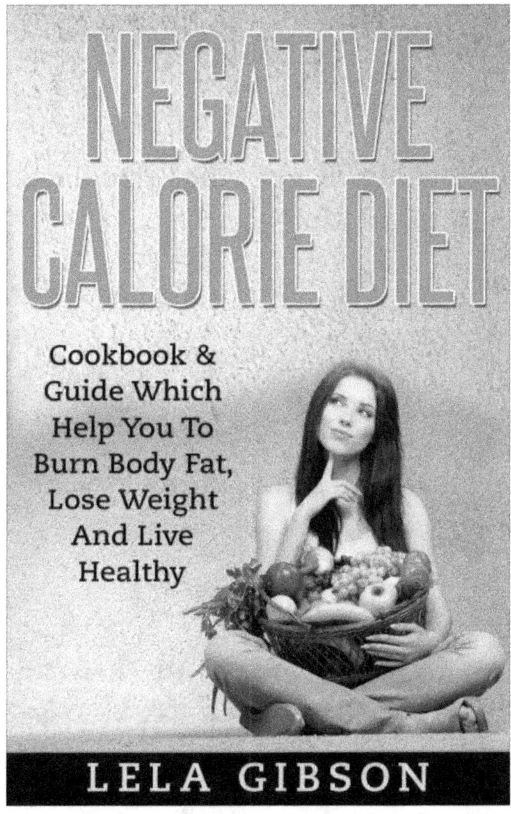

Check out the rest of Negative Calorie Diet on Amazon.

Go to: http://amzn.to/2mkjJuh

Check Out My Other Books

Below you'll find some of my other popular books that are popular on Amazon and Kindle as well.

Alternatively, you can visit my author page on Amazon to see other work done by me.

20 Easy And Fast Diet Tips For Losing Weight – An Easy-To-Follow Weight Loss Guide

Belly Diet: The Zero Belly Diet Step-By-Step Guide Which Will Help You To Lose Your Belly And Enjoy Your Flat Belly

Anti-Inflammatory Diet Guide – The Guide To Reduce Inflammation And Live A Healthy Life Without Pain

Dash Diet: Cookbook For Weight Loss With Action Plan And Easy Recipes

Clean Eating: Cookbook And Guide To Restore Your Body's Natural Balance And Eat Healthy

63

Negative Calorie Diet: Cookbook & Guide Which Help You To Burn Body Fat, Lose Weight And Live Healthy

www.ingramcontent.com/pod-product-compliance
Lightning Source LLC
Chambersburg PA
CBHW070046260726
48658CB00002B/765